I0441005

Fitness at Workplace

How to Improve Health & Productivity at Your Workplace to Achieve Peak Performance

By

Jillian Michael

© 2014 by BookStage

Digital Edition

This book is licensed for your personal enjoyment
only. This book may not be re-sold or given away to
other people. If you would like to share this book with
another person, please purchase an additional copy
for each recipient. If you're reading this book and did
not purchase it, or it was not purchased for your use
only, then please purchase your own copy. Thank you
for respecting the hard work of this author.

All Rights Reserved. No part of this book may be
reproduced in any form or by any electronic or
mechanical means including information storage and
retrieval systems without permission in writing from
the publisher, except by a reviewer who may quote
brief passages in a review.

The content of this book has been reviewed for
accuracy. However, the author and publisher disclaim
any liability for any damages, losses, or injuries that
may result from the use or misuse of any product or
information presented herein. It is the purchaser's
responsibility to read and follow all instructions and
warnings on all product labels.

For information, please contact the author at
info@bookstage.net

Table of Contents

Chapter 1

Importance of Fitness at Workplace

A decade ago, requesting your employer to consider implementing a fitness at workplace strategy would have led to criticism, censure, and even loss of job. This is probably how your superiors would have discussed the issue.

Superior 1

"He suggested we not just allow but actually encourage employees to exercise in the office."

Superior 2

"What? Exercise in the office! Is he/she serious about work? Does he/she think we are running a gym?"

Superior 1

"Just my thoughts too. Let's just get rid of him/her before he/she comes up with other weird ideas."

Bottom line

Office was for work. Not for leisurely activities like jogging, calisthenics, and exercising. Do your work. Earn your pay. And if you want to exercise, join a gym.

Today, such a suggestion would probably result in a pat on your back along with your photo on the notice board for

"Best Suggestion Of The Month", "Most Sincere Employee", "Potential Future CEO", and so on.

So, what has changed? Why is the idea of fitness at workplace gaining currency? Why are employees, employers, and even the authorities encouraging this concept?

From the employee's i.e. your perspective, exercising in your office makes complete sense. According to the 2012 American Time Use Survey by the Bureau of Labor, an average individual between the age group of 25 to 54 years spends 8.8 hours doing work and work related activities. In 2009, this figure was 7.9 hours. Your working day isn't getting any shorter.

According to the 2012 data, excluding work and sleep, we are left with just 7.5 hours for other activities including eating, doing household chores, caring for your loved ones and so on. Where is the time or motivation to focus on fitness?

In such a scenario, having a 30-minute exercise break at work can make a huge difference.

- No more guilt when having a donut? Check.

- Higher energy levels at work? Check.

- Better camaraderie with colleagues? Check.

- Better home life due to less stress, more productivity, and higher energy levels? Check.

Sounds great, right?

For employers, healthier employees means less absenteeism, more productivity, reduced compensation claims, cheaper medical insurance, and fewer instances of loss of valuable employees with years of experience to lifestyle diseases. And of course, fitness at workplace makes for great PR as well.

For the authorities, government, and nation as a whole, awareness about fitness will be a gift that will keep on giving. The obesity epidemic abates, productive citizens don't die at the prime of their lives, strain on the medical infrastructure will come down, and as awareness about fitness percolates down to the kids, the army will not have to deal with the problem of converting obese and unfit youngsters into lean, trim, and strong soldiers.

Chapter 2

What Your Fitness At Workplace Strategy Must Cover?

What is worse than not having a fitness at office strategy? Having a poorly designed strategy that causes more harm than good. Whether it is a routine to be executed use in your cubicle or a strategy for all your coworkers, it is very important to have a comprehensive and effective fitness strategy. Only then will you and your office enjoy sustainable and consistent results.

The first and most important aspect is general physical fitness. A sedentary lifestyle involving sitting in front of the computer for hours together can wreak havoc with your general physical health. Avoiding weight gain is next to impossible even if you try to avoid fatty and sugary foods.

An effective fitness strategy must begin with improving physical fitness. A stroll around the office, a quick session of aerobics and calisthenics, or repeatedly climbing a flight of stairs—there are innumerable options that help you exert your muscles and bring your body back into shape.

Apart from general physical fitness, the routine should also cover steps and activities designed to prevent occupational diseases and ailments. Wrist and forearm exercises can minimize risk of Repetitive Strain Injury for employees who spend a lot of time typing on the keyboard.

Those who spend hours staring at the computer screen would benefit from neck exercises aimed at preventing Spondylitis and other such problems. Yoga and breathing exercises may help those exposed to dust, smoke, and industrial pollutants. Simply take a look at ailments and illnesses that led to compensation claims in your office and try to come up with an exercise regimen to minimize such occurrences.

Focusing solely on physical fitness is not a smart move. Stress, tension, suppressed emotions, frustration, and feeling of incompetence—the average office worker runs the risk of suffering from many mental ailments as well. Ailments of the mind are tougher to diagnose and impossible to treat through medicines alone.

A holistic fitness strategy that strengthens the body and mind of the employee can prove to be a worthwhile investment in the long run. To sum it up, your personal or group fitness strategy should cover the following:

- Custom-designed to meet the unique requirements of your office.
- Multiple options ranging from training with weights to running on the treadmill to yoga.
- Equal emphasis on physical and mental fitness.
- A sensible approach that integrates fitness routines into the functioning of the office.

Chapter 3

Formal Fitness At Workplace Programs

Until half a decade ago, corporations and employers viewed fitness as a personal decision that did not belong in the office. Today, 92% of companies employing 200 persons or more have a formal wellness program in place. So, what has changed? And how does this change affect you?

The National Health and Nutrition Examination Survey 2009-10 found that 35% of adults above the age of 20 years were obese. Now, obesity can lead to a whole range of diseases and complications ranging from diabetes, blood pressure, cardio-vascular problems and arthritis.

A 2007 study by the Duke University discovered that obese workers were twice as likely to file compensation claims and would incur seven times higher medical costs. Further, loss of work days due to work injury or work illness would be 13 times higher for obese workers as compared to fit workers.

Medical insurance costs more for unfit and obese people as they are more likely to fall ill. Companies that hire unfit persons will have to spend more money on medical insurance. Finally, companies will also have to spend on training replacements for those who quit due to recurring health problems.

Bluntly put, the cost of implementing a fitness or wellness program at work outweighed the costs of treating it as a personal decision of the employees. Hence, keep in mind that your employer is not doing you a favor by implementing a fitness program. Rather, they are doing themselves a favor and you are definitely entitled to receive their support and assistance in improving your fitness and health.

How Employer Fitness & Wellness Programs Work?

The programs can be broadly categorized as:

a. Health Risk Assessment & Awareness Programs

Your employer pays for health checkups and medical tests to help you learn more about your fitness levels. Your employer pays for activities like health checkups, Body Mass analysis, Lipid Profile tests, Diabetes & Blood Pressure tests, Heart checkups, Awareness seminars, Counseling sessions, and lectures by fitness gurus. The logic is to help you become aware of the risks and costs of being unfit and encourage you to focus on your fitness.

b. Disease Management Programs

These programs are designed for employees who have begun to suffer the consequences of a sedentary lifestyle. The employer chips in to minimize impact of lifestyle diseases on the employee's productivity. These programs normally cover medical intervention, holistic remedies, and counseling sessions.

Some employers may have specific programs for obese employees or workers addicted to tobacco, alcohol, or substance abuse.

c. Fitness & Exercise Programs

In these programs, the employer actively contributes to help you and your colleagues improve your fitness.

These programs include:
- Setting up a gym at office.
- Offering subsidized memberships as a perk
- Providing wellness facilities combined with individual targets. Successful employees get incentives while laggards are penalized.
- Providing a wide range of options ranging from treadmill at the office to sponsoring participation in marathons and triathlons and allowing employees to choose their preferred fitness routine.
- Establishing benchmarks for different age-groups and adopting a carrot/stick policy to encourage compliance.
- Weight-loss centric programs as opposed to general fitness solutions.

Now, each option has its own set of pros and cons. General assessment and awareness programs will help you learn more about the impact of a sedentary lifestyle. You will be free to choose an approach that suits your body without any employer intervention. However, the onus of improving your fitness is on you and you probably won't get a lot of help from the organization.

Disease management programs are great for those who are struggling to cope with lifestyle ailments. However, this is a rather pessimistic approach where focus is on curing rather than preventing diseases arising out of poor fitness.

Fitness programs with active participation by the employer can make a huge difference. A gym at office will mean you can include a 30-minute run in your office routine. A cycling track or rock climbing wall in the office premises can make work a lot more fun. Subsidized gym memberships don't hurt either.

However, the biggest disadvantage of such a setup is that you become accountable to your employers for rapid loss of weight. Instead of focusing on the quality of improvement, the organization may become obsessed with pounds lost and inches trimmed. Paying penalties for not losing weight as fast as your colleague can be very embarrassing and frustrating.

Like all other HR ideas, the fitness program may too become a cause for stress and tension as opposed to a cure. Suggesting improvements or modifications to the program can become a big headache as it may involve going through multiple layers of corporate bureaucracy.

How Should You Proceed?

Well, the smartest option is to participate wholeheartedly in the program setup by your employer to enjoy its benefits. However, it is important to keep the final goal in mind. The purpose of fitness programs is to improve health and fitness. You will have to, through individual or collective efforts, ensure the program does not end up as a formality.

All said and done, it does not make sense to be too cynical about such formal programs. There has been a drastic change in the mindset of employers in the past decade and this setup is only going to get better. Working out with your colleagues can provide more motivation as compared to working out alone in the gym. Informal competitions with a rival department can add that extra bit of zing to your workout regimen. And finally, you will have more time and energy when interacting with your spouse and kids back home—a real blessing.

And if it doesn't work, you always have the option of climbing flights of stairs and doing crunches on your office chair to enjoy a good workout during office hours.

Chapter 4

Workplaces Without Formal Programs

It has become fashionable for corporations, big and small, to speak in favor of wellness programs at workplaces. However, while big companies are walking the talk, small businesses are yet to embrace this concept fully.

A 2012 survey conducted by the National Small Business Association indicates that while 93% of small businesses were in favor of having an employee health program, just 22% were actually offering such a program to their workers. Data on the website of the Centers for Disease Control and Prevention indicates that businesses lose around $226 billion dollars every year due to productivity losses caused by personal and family health problems.

Don't be surprised if your employer is not inclined to provide any real support for an employee wellness or fitness program. Be prepared to argue your case to convince your employer. The best option is to adopt a twin-pronged approach where you try to convince your employer and take steps to implement an informal and unofficial fitness routine for yourself and your co-workers.

Convincing Your Employer

Times have been tough and one can't really blame small business owners for their reluctance to embrace ideas that involve extra expenditure. However, spending money on a wellness program is not an expense; it is an investment.

There have been innumerable surveys and studies conducted to analyze the impact of poor employee health on the profits of the organization. Use the data to build a coherent case. Check out success stories that highlight the monetary and other benefits of having a healthier and happier workforce.

It is very important to approach the top guy in your office with your idea. Sending it through normal channels of communication may lead to the idea being buried even before it reaches your CEO. Don't focus on monetary benefits alone. From better camaraderie amongst employees to the immense PR opportunities that such programs afford, make sure you cover all facets and aspects of the program.

Finally, don't try to bully your employer into approving the deal. It is not just a question of allocation of funds. Allowing employees to focus on fitness as a part of their normal work life requires a huge shift in work culture. Hence, make sure you come up with an alternative plan that does not require any financial investment from your employer.

Requesting the employer to grant a 30-minute exercise break where employees will exercise on equipment purchased through group contributions may be a great way to convince a boss reluctant to spend money on the idea. The employer may change his or her mind once the program begins and the benefits, monetary and non-monetary, start accruing.

Proceeding without Employer Support

The trick to implementing a workplace fitness strategy without contribution from the employer is to keep it simple, cheap, and effective. Get a hoop installed on the wall to encourage employees to have a short basketball match to exercise the muscles.

Climbing stairs to burn calories can be very boring. Get your co-workers to join you in this task. Use the countdown timer in your smartphone to time the performance of each individual. Introducing some competitive sprit can have a very positive effect on the enthusiasm of your co-workers.

Have measurable goals. Losing a few pounds of extra flab through office exercises sounds a lot more exciting than targeting general health and fitness. Until you convince your employer to support a full-fledged program, make sure you focus on short-term targets that can be achieved without complications.

Informal Program—Blessing in Disguise

While a formal program will have a defined structure with health assessment, disease prevention, and fitness strategies, an informal regimen has its own unique benefits and advantages. You will have the freedom of setting your own goals. You can demarcate exercises and routines to be done as a group and will have complete freedom to include whatever you want in your individual routine.

Secondly, the question of ROI will just not arise. A formal program with its budget and funding will lead to questions about return on the investment. Instead of a voluntary self-help venture, the routine will get converted into one of those things that you are compulsorily required to do at your workplace.

Thirdly, you can be a lot more creative and include unorthodox activities as well. Trying out kick boxing under a formal program can be next to impossible with the company worrying about injuries, compensation claims, and a host of other issues. In a routine agreed upon by all the workers, trying out something new will involve nothing more than the free consent of the participants.

Start From Your Cubicle & Work Your Way Outside

What exercises can you do sitting in your chair in your cubicle? Aisles are great for stretching your body. The staircase is a good way to tone your thighs and legs with some cardio training. The lobby or the porch is a great place to stroll, get some fresh air, and relax your mind. The parking lot can be used for aerobics.

The trick to coming up with an effective routine is to start with those exercises that can be done in the cubicle and work your way out to the front gate. This gives you a lot of scope for variety, which can prove very beneficial once your muscles start tiring.

Informal Programs May Be The Way To Go

While big companies are investing in wellness programs at workplaces, the jury is still out on its effectiveness. More often than not, the purpose underlying the program gets diluted as managers convert the program into a formality.

In such a scenario, informal programs with a high level of employee participation and minimal employer interference may well be the way to proceed. You could consider trying this option before proceeding ahead with a full-fledged formal program run by your management.

Chapter 5

Inexpensive Ideas To Make Workplace Fitness More Enjoyable

Let's be honest—exercising can hardly be described as the most exciting and entertaining activity in the world. Pushing your body beyond the limits of your endurance requires a lot of willpower and motivation. Combining a rigorous fitness regimen with a hectic office schedule can become a nightmare where you rush to meet impossible deadlines with tired limbs, cramped muscles, and aching body parts.

Exercising in your office will be very tough, especially in the initial phase. This is why you should focus on coming up with the most creative and innovative ways to make workplace fitness more fun. You don't have the option of quitting; just imagine what your snarky colleagues would say? Instead, just utilize these fun ideas to make office fitness routines more fun and enjoyable.

An Office Fitness Newsletter

An e-newsletter providing updates about the latest changes to the regimen can be a simple and effective way to improve motivation and encourage participation. Colleagues can be encouraged to share tips, ideas, and suggestions, along with information about the monetary and other benefits of exercising in the office.

A newsletter can prove very useful in lending a formal appeal to an informal program designed and implemented by the office staff. In case of a formal program with the involvement of the management, the newsletter can serve as a useful channel of communication as well.

E-newsletter can have videos and images explaining the right way to perform tough exercises. It can serve as a customized tutorial for those who are struggling to match the pace of the regimen.

Fitness Contests

Add a pinch of competitive spirit to ensure the buzz surrounding the wellness program hits the roof. Who is the fittest amongst them all? Who has the strongest muscles, the most stamina, and the slimmest waist? Truth we told, we all compete with our colleagues and coworkers.

From arriving on time to meeting monthly targets— a certain amount of competition is always good for productivity. From cheesy certificates to a honorable mention on the notice board, you can come up with numerous award ideas to encourage people to work out harder and get fit faster.

Levying Fines to Finance Equipment Purchase

Those who perform poorly in the contests or those who fail to meet fitness targets can be asked to contribute to a common pool. The fund can then be used to buy fitness equipments like fitness cycles, treadmills, or even pedometers.

Apart from encouraging people to work out harder, such a system will ensure you have all the necessary equipment and accessories for a full-fledged workout. Or, the fund can be used to finance healthy snacks, which will only serve to improve the overall health and fitness of the office staff.

Just make sure the amount is not too high and that the fines are paid in good spirit. It should be seen as an innovative fund-raising idea as opposed to a punishment or penalty.

Indoor Sporting Arenas

Basketball hoop placed at strategic locations throughout the office can help sports enthusiasts try some one-on-one competition to burn the extra calories and work stress without a lot of effort. A boxing bag is ideal for those who reducing flab through boxing sessions. Even a Frisbee will help improve reflexes and focus.

You can take the sting out of exercising by opting for indoor sports. Of course, safety is a big issue but a workable arrangement can be done considering that burning calories is the primary objective here.

Cycle to Work

Who says office fitness programs should involve exercising in the office only? Cycling to work is a great way to start the day. A relaxed ride back home after a tough day will help get rid of stress. Cycling together in a group will help mask the effort and enhance the overall quality of experience. It will make for great PR as well when people see employees of a firm burning calories and protecting the environment by cycling to work.

Invite Suggestions from Spouses/Kids

Exercising at work can be very exhausting in the initial phase. It is important to obtain support of spouses and kids of all the employees. A great way to make them feel a part of the program is to invite creative low-budget exercise ideas and suggestions from them. Even if the ideas don't work, the goodwill that this gesture will generate will help overcome the initial tough phase.

Health Lunches & Healthy Recipe Contests

What is the point of participating in an office fitness program if you are going to consume greasy lunches and snacks filled with sugar and carbs during breaks? Try to inculcate healthy eating habits. Have a healthy dish contest to get people to contribute healthy ways of making tasty dishes.

Such an activity will ensure the benefits of regular exercises are not lost due to unhealthy eating.

Healthy Snacks & Drinks in the Office Vending Machine

This is just an extension of getting your coworkers to eat healthier food. Including healthy snacks in the cafeteria menu or making packaged fruit juices available as an alternative to tea and coffee can prove very beneficial in the long run.

Wellness & Fitness Buddies

Ever heard of the good cop bad cop routine? Well, you can create fitness teams consisting of two employees working in different departments. The buddy's job is to lend a hand to ease the workload and to help ensure the fitness regimen stays on track. The buddy system can be very helpful in improving team work and staying motivated.

Avatar-type Fitness journals

Do you remember how characters in the movie Avatar made video journals of their experiences? You can encourage people to maintain a diary, a blog, or even a video journal of their experiences and improvements.

Such journals can be shared with others in the office to ensure everybody understands the impact of the wellness program on their coworkers. What is more, such entries, posts, and videos will look great in your department's annual yearbook.

Children's Games

Ever observed children playing games? Their games are simple, involve a lot of running and physical activity, and are invariably accompanied with lots of laughter. Try playing tag with your entire office team. Sure, some people may find it childish but you will find it to be a great stress buster. Simply teaming up with others and running around will help you burn calories. The joy of playing like kids again—that is an additional benefit.

Fitness-Centric Treasure Hunt

Organize a treasure hunt where people have to perform specific exercises and physical activities to get the next clue. As prizes, you can offer preferential access to the fitness equipment or food vouchers for healthy food in the cafeteria.

You can have one-on-one contests where the first person to complete 20 pushups in one minute progresses to the next clue or group activities where the team gets the next clue when every team member completes a specific exercise.

Such games will ensure wellness and fitness activities are associated with fun and joy rather than pain and discomfort.

Dance & Music

Just let yourself go on the dance floor. Burn the flab by doing the Cha Cha Cha. Dancing is a very effective form of cardio exercises where you can burn calories without even realizing that you are working out.

It is a great option for stress release and will be a good way to loosen up and relax after a tough day full of meetings and deadlines.

Video Games

This may sound odd but new-age video games can help you improve your fitness. Consoles with motion sensing technology convert actions in real life into video game movements. A racing game will require you to hop at the same spot in front of the console. If you are looking for something really radical, you can opt for Wii or Kinect games where you get to work out when playing your favorite video game in the office.

Chapter 6

Risks & Pitfalls of Fitness at Workplace Programs

Fitness at workplace programs may seem like the next best thing after the wheel and sliced break for a person struggling to focus on work, home, and fitness at the same time. However, this does not mean such programs don't have any drawbacks or pitfalls. There are some risks that you must recognize and work around to ensure your individual or group program offers consistent and sustainable results.

All Hype But No Action

It is easy to express support or admiration for such programs. However, it can be very difficult to actually start exercising at work. It requires a huge change in mindset and work culture. Even if your boss supports such an idea, getting people from diverse backgrounds to work together towards a personal issue like fitness can be very tough.

Make sure your idea does not get stuck at the planning stage. Don't wait for the perfect moment. Start exercising to ensure the idea gets momentum. Expanding the program will be a lot easier once it becomes a part of your work culture.

What About The Money?

A full-fledged program will involve some unavoidable expenses. Of course, you can skip fancy equipment and accessories and keep things simple in the beginning to avoid funding issues. However, as the idea spreads and as the scale of the program expands, you may find it impossible to avoid expenditure.

Your colleagues may be cool with using the stairs as a form of cardio and doing aerobics and yoga in the conference room. However, disease management, health assessment, and preventive checkups will cost money. This is why you should consider involving the management as soon as possible.

Management's Hidden Agenda

Which bring us to the next risk. You and your colleagues may be keen on losing weight and enjoying improved health. However, your management need not share the same goals. This is not to say that your employers are evil or wrong. They may have a different perspective, one that involves higher productivity at lower costs.

The question of penalizing people for not meeting fitness goals does not arise in an informal program. However, a formal program with significant investment may involve rigid goals that may bring penalties, fines, or even censure to the laggards.

Further, the management may seek to convert the exercise into a PR spectacle. This may not be a bad idea as long as the regimen does not end up as an elaborate advertising campaign that offers no real benefits to the employees.

Injuries and Interpersonal Conflicts

Everybody wants to be healthy and fit. However, this common goal may not be enough when you are working in a group. Attitude problems, ego differences, and different thinking styles can easily lead to interpersonal conflict.

Who gets to the lead the program? The fittest? The one who came up with this idea? The management's choice? Or, the richest? How to handle snarky comments from those who are fitter than others? How to prevent jealousies or work-related conflicts from becoming an issue?

And then there are injuries. Will the management be liable for claims arising out of fitness program injuries? What if it is an informal program? Who pays? What if the management decides to punish employees for performing exercises that led to injuries?

From the human and interpersonal angle to the financial and medical angle, make sure you consider all the facets and aspects before proceeding ahead with the program.

Chapter 7

Office Fitness Program: Beyond Conventional Exercises

There was a time when physical fitness was measured by the size of one's waist and other body parts. A slim figure was considered fit while a flabby body was considered unfit. There is no doubt that being overweight is an indicator of poor fitness. However, good health and fitness involves a lot more than having bulging biceps and slim waistlines. Hence, make sure you focus on real health and fitness that involves something more than physical appearances.

A desk worker has nothing to gain from having bulging biceps and a six-pack abs. A flexible, fit, and active body combined with a peaceful mind will be more beneficial as far as job performance is concerned. Hence, consider the following options over and above the conventional exercises that form a part of the office fitness regimen.

Yoga

Over the years, yoga has become a very popular fitness option and you would do well to include this in your office wellness program. For starters, yoga is suitable for people of all ages, which can prove very beneficial in an office with employees of all ages. Secondly, the yoga postures are primarily aimed at improving fitness and general health. There are numerous sets of yoga postures designed for improving flexibility and dexterity in different muscles.

Hence, from asanas or postures for general health to asanas for diabetes, back pain, joint pain, or repetitive strain injury, you have a lot of choice and options. The best part is that the asanas can be combined with stretching and warm up exercises to enhance the overall efficacy of the exercise regimen.

Pilates

Pilates consists of a series of exercises and movements designed to strengthen the body and mind. Like Yoga, Pilates too adopts a comprehensive approach and treats the body and the mind as two sides of the same coin.

Pilates is all about concentration, control, centering, smooth flow of body movements, precision in movements and actions, combined with breathing control. The basic logic underlying Pilates seems very similar to Yoga but the postures and methods differ. This can prove very helpful for those who are not comfortable with Yoga.

Pilates and Yoga have postures and exercises that can be performed in your seat as well. This means that you can have a comprehensive workout without even getting up from your desk. If you don't have the support of your employers or if your office lacks space, then these exercise options that don't require a lot of space can prove very useful.

Meditation

Along with exercises and activities that strengthen your body, you should also include ways and means to increase mental strength. Lack of exercise, a sedentary lifestyle, and unhealthy diets are significant reasons for ill health and fitness but there is no denying that stress acts as the force multiplier that causes significant damage to the body and mind.

Stress cannot be tackled through physical activities alone. Of course, working as a group and developing camaraderie can help but the simplest and most effective way to tackle stress is meditation. From listening to soothing music in your cubicle, having discussions on spiritual and religious topics, to simply closing your eyes and relaxing your body and mind—you have a lot of choice as far as the form of meditation is concerned.

While Yoga, Pilates, Aerobics, or Calisthenics can lead to injuries if done improperly, there are no negative side effects of meditation. Just choose the approach that you are most comfortable with and use it to reduce your stress levels.

Healthier Office Lunches & Snacks

What you eat has a huge impact on your health. Improving the health quotient of office lunches can have a very significant effect on fitness levels. Starting with the diet will create the right atmosphere in the office for the implementation of the wellness program. You will find your employer and colleagues amenable to an enhanced fitness regimen once the concept of healthy eating becomes a part of your office culture.

It is a misconception that healthy foodstuffs cost more and are more cumbersome to prepare. The cost of healthy and organic food will definitely be lower than the increased medical insurance premiums that your employer has to bear. As far as preparation is concerned, it is a matter of opinion and one has to consider the overall benefits before taking a call on this aspect.

Conclusion

There is no limit to the various alternatives or additions to conventional exercises. Just make sure you don't end up with a regimen that involves trying different options without sticking to even a single one. A week of Yoga may seem very enjoyable if it breaks the monotony of aerobics and cardio exercises. Pilates can force you to step outside your comfort zone by doing something new. Reverting to the cardio routine may give the feeling of doing some 'real' exercises as compared to the Yoga postures.

There is no right or wrong here. What matters is that the components of your office wellness strategy must serve its purpose—to help you improve your overall health and fitness.

About the Author

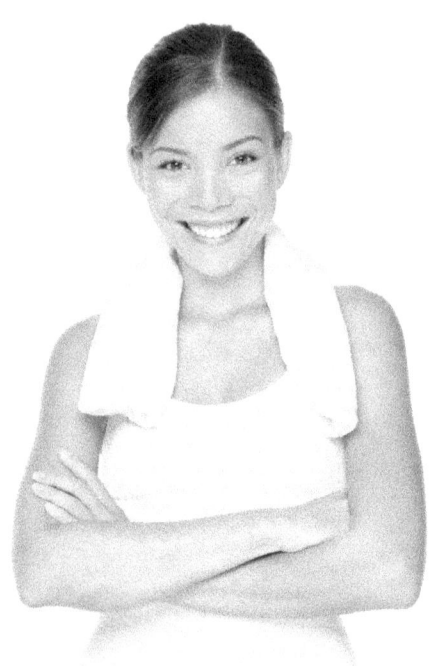

With 15 years of experience in the fitness industry, Jillian Michael has witnessed the transformation of attitudes and mindset towards health and fitness in our society over the past two decades. A regular contributor of articles and columns to newspapers and fitness magazines, Jillian has formulated effective and sustainable fitness at workplace strategies for employers and employees alike. She lives in New Jersey with her husband, daughter, and two pet dogs.

References

- http://www.fitness-nutrition-weightloss.com
- http://www.cpihr.com
- http://www.cdc.gov
- http://www.ccohs.ca
- http://www.livestrong.com
- http://www.dol.gov
- http://corporate.dukemedicine.org
- http://www.benefitspro.com
- http://wellnessproposals.com

www.ingramcontent.com/pod-product-compliance
Lightning Source LLC
Chambersburg PA
CBHW070133290526
45789CB00005B/2229